Shattering the Illusion of Disease

The 7 Steps to Reclaiming you Perfect Health

PETER D. ADAMS

Visionary Publishing

Shattering the Illusion of Disease

Published by Visionary Publishing

Published in the United States of America

ISBN-13: 978-0-692-04265-6

CONTENTS

DEDICATION

This book is dedicated to YOU,
THE MOST IMPORTANT PERSON IN
THE WORLD...

FOREWORD

No matter what you may be experiencing at this moment, perfect health is honestly only a thought away. Everything that you are experiencing results directly from all the thoughts, beliefs, emotions, and fears you have ever held in your mind. The summation of these things which you have run through your mind and held on to is creating your reality.

Stopping the runaway train which runs on fear is simple: remove the fuel source. You do this by consciously changing the thoughts you think until you have changed your entire belief system. Once your belief system has changed for good, what you will then experience is perfect health, happiness, and abundance in your life.

However, if you are not willing to do what is needed to re-wire your mind, you will see the condition of poor health stay with your experience. Perfect health and healing is an internal process, and all the doctors and drugs in the world will not get you there if your mind believes in the polar opposite.

As you will see, everything you experience on the outside was first created on the inside. Therefore, everything that you are experiencing can be reversed and eliminated through changing the thoughts and beliefs you hold in your mind. You have the power to replace a lifetime of sickness with perfect health being your reality for now and the future. If you are ready for a massive positive change in your life, then let us begin...

———

CHAPTER 1

HEALTHCARE INC.

Before we talk about a return to perfect health, I want to spend some time explaining our health care system. Understanding how the "system" works and what the motivations are between different parties that make up the system will help you with any decision you need to make about your health and ultimately the care you choose or do not choose to receive.

The first thing you must understand is that healthcare is a BUSINESS first, all else second. The primary focus of any healthcare provider, whether it is your primary care physician, a specialist, or a facility, is to make as much profit as humanly possible! If that sounds a little simplistic, it is not. How they make insane profits is due in a great part to the lack of information and transparency shared with the public. The industry refers to the policies they have in place and follow as being "trade secrets." The only reason they want to keep their pricing secret is because if the public knew what was going on, they would be up in arms!

You probably think that I have harsh views on healthcare, and you would be correct. I worked on the business side of the "machine" as both an analyst and as a director of finance. In total, I spent six years working in the business, and what I learned was enough to make me want to dismantle the complete system and start over from scratch. The level of greed I have seen and experienced behind closed doors would sound so far-fetched that it could not be true. Rather than talk in abstracts, let me give you an example of something I personally witnessed.

Back when I was the Director of Finance for a practice management company in Florida, which oversaw a large group of physicians and managed the business side for them. On this particular day, which I will never forget for as long as I live, I attended a board meeting to discuss the prior period's financial results. After the board meeting was adjourned, the statewide Chief Financial Officer and I met with an eye surgeon behind closed doors. The eye surgeon did not feel he was being compensated enough for his services. We explained to him that our company did not set the rates of compensation for specialists; instead, they were set by the physicians who founded the organization which he was a part of. He said, "**You know I would probably do a better job operating on your grandmother if I was not concerned with thinking about my level of compensation while I am in surgery.**"

I could not believe that he said that. I was speechless. On the drive back to our office, the CFO and I were dumbstruck. Did we really hear that? A doctor would never say anything like that. Right?? He said that, and money was the only reason he ever got in to the field of medicine.

Recently, there was a physician caught in Vail, for intentionally misdiagnosing people as having multiple sclerosis when they did not have it. Treating this "incurable disease" then leads to a lifetime of treatments that are incredibly expensive, which then nets the physician a lifetime of income. Unfortunately, all the people he deliberately misdiagnosed and ruined years of their lives never got their day in court and received no compensation as the doctor had let his malpractice insurance policy lapse. Because there was no insurance company to sue for a large settlement, the trial attorneys never pursued the case as there was not going to be a big payday for anyone.

The doctor lost his right to practice medicine in the State of , but if this doesn't make your head spin, he is now actively practicing medicine on the Palm Coast of Florida!

The medical profession does everything that they can do to keep these occurrences out of the media. No one, including me, knows how many of these extreme cases there are, but it is enough to make you wonder how common it is. What is far more common are procedures and therapies being done every day, which are unnecessary and are only being done to bring in more revenue.

Managed Care

Managed care is a term you probably have heard of before, especially if you live in the . Managed care can best be described as the competition for dollars in the health care marketplace. To keep it simple, you buy health insurance and you pay a certain amount each month to an insurance company, which makes you a "customer" in their eyes. The insurance company wants to take in as much premium from you as possible and pay out as little as they can for health care services. One way they do this is to have high up-front deductibles and/or expensive co-pays that you must pay before the insurance company spends any money. By doing this, they keep you from seeking services from providers because it is simply too expensive.

Another far less obvious way they keep you from spending "their money" is to require you to pick out a doctor to be your Primary Care Provider, or "PCP" for short. Once you have selected a Primary Care Provider, you are then considered on their "panel", which means you are a customer and that the PCP will receive financial compensation each month based upon your age and sex directly from the insurance company. For the PCP to make serious money, their model is to create the largest panel possible, and then to see as few patients as they can. If you have ever wondered why it is that when you call your doctor's office and tell them you are sick, and they tell you the earliest they can see you is in seven weeks, that is the reason. If you feel better over the next seven weeks, they have successfully kept you from spending "their money," as the only way to access non-emergency care is through coordinating it through your Primary Care Provider. If you try to get care without going to your PCP first, they will refuse to pay, and then you are stuck with the bill. Sometimes it doesn't go as planned for the insurance company; let's say that a block of tests are done and you get admitted in to a hospital.

This is where the competition for dollars gets a little intense. The providers of health care services are paid through a system known as Fee for Service or "FFS" for short. The more services they can provide, be they necessary or not, the more they will get paid. They will perform all the services they can under the guise of providing you with great care. Their entire goal is to never lose you as a "customer" and to keep you coming back to them for as long as they can. The insurance companies know and hate this, as they know they are on the hook for the bill unless they can find a loophole to pass it back on to you. That is why you will notice that anytime someone is admitted to the hospital, the insurance company will immediately assign them a case manager, whose role is to get the patient out of the hospital as soon as possible and to have the least number of services or procedures done to the customer.

One of the real challenges in the way the health care system works is that the providers, let's say a hospital, cut a deal with the insurance company and the hospital gets paid on what is known in the industry as "a percentage of billed charges." The standard deal is 70% of what the hospital has charged the customer for their hospital stay, and that is what the insurance company will pay the hospital. I worked for the largest for-profit hospital company in the United States, and our goal at the hospital was to increase our net profit by 15% each year. In the hospital, there is a "price list" that contains every service and product that the hospital offers and is known as the "charge master." We essentially made up our own prices we charged and then increased them every year by 15% or more. When you hear about someone getting charged $100 for a single aspirin tablet, it is true, and that is the perfect example of a price we "made up" and then charged the customer for. The insurance company is just a middleman, so they raise the prices of their premiums by 15% or more each year so they can maintain their profit margin.

On the Government side of health care with Medicare & Medicaid, the Government sets the price which they will pay for anything and everything. Which is good because if they didn't, the taxes we all would pay to support the system would not be sustainable.

Big Pharma

A discussion about our healthcare industry would not be complete without talking about the pharmaceuticals industry (aka Big Pharma) which manufactures the drugs that our society is told they must have. Big Pharma makes incredible profits and the prices they charge are insane in relation to the costs involved in research and development. Their motivation is to get someone else to pay for the research from grants or other initiatives possibly funded by taxpayers, and then to turn around when the drug is ready and gouge the consumer for all its worth. Better yet, *let's get you a prescription for something that you must take every day for "the rest of your life!"*

Lobbyists

Every one of the major players in the health care industry knows how important it is to control the politicians and their decision-making powers. That is why there are so many lobbyists representing the interest of these companies. That is why the Affordable Health-care Act turned out how it did. The entire document was drafted by Healthcare Inc.'s lobbyists, and it essentially locks in a profit for the insurance companies no matter what happens. If you want another example of how our politicians are beholden to the lobbyists and the money, just watch two hours of television and notice that most of all the commercials are for pharmaceuticals. Only two countries in the world allow drug companies to do "direct to consumer advertising," and they are the United States and New Zealand. The reason no other countries allow this advertising is because they know about the power of suggestion. The advertising creates the suggestion, "You better see your doctor as you probably have _____ disease," and just from that suggestion, people begin to experience symptoms which they have created in their mind, and now it is showing up in their experience as a direct result of the commercial. For politicians, I guess it just means they will do whatever it takes to get elected and stay in office, and if a couple of people die along the way, no one will notice.

The Power of Suggestion

Marketing in healthcare is all about the power of suggestion, and to sum it up in one word, that word would be "FEAR." They are honestly trying to convince you that if you are not already sick, then just wait a little while and you will be. Now that you know about the Fee for Service model, you realize that health care providers must perform some procedures or tests on you or they won't get paid. The perfect example of this is what I call the "Jiffy Lube" checkup. Back when I lived in Florida, I used to bring my car in for an oil change at the local Jiffy Lube store. Without fail, every time I stopped by to get the $19.95 advertised oil change, before long I would be approached by an employee who would have a tray of various liquids showing what was pristine on one side, and what the liquids looked like from my car. Fortunately for me, when I was growing up, I learned how to maintain the family automobile, so I know when I am being lied to by these guys. It got so bad that over time I would just give them a hard time when they tried selling me services like:

- a radiator flush and conditioning service.

- scraping the oil stuck on the inside of my

oil pan from driving over 3,000 between oil changes.

- replacing my air filter for only $5\times$ more than I could buy one and do it myself in one minute.

- complete transmission conditioning package which included replacing the filter and the transmission fluid.

The car at the time needed none of these services as it was new, and they were just trying to sell me things I didn't need to make more money themselves. Now, I want you to think about the last time you had a checkup with your doctor. How many tests did they run? Even though you said that you felt great and had excellent health? I am sure that they didn't take your word for it, which then leads to later visits, follow-ups, etc. The worst example of this that I have seen repeatedly is when healthcare providers get their hands on older "customers." It is almost like once you get Dr. Smith on your calendar you never get him off it. Every time you see him, they set the next appointment for you to come back, and the process is repeated for the rest of your life.

To give you a perfect example of the power of suggestion, let me use the example of "flu shots" which are given out to senior citizens. The entire marketing idea almost seems as though it comes out of the middle ages, and the storyline is about how many people die each year from getting the flu. The flu shot they give you is an injection which contains the influenza virus. I know people who have gotten a flu shot every year, and every year they have gotten sick with the flu afterward. Do you think that is "coincidence?" Now that they are sick, they must spend more of their money on doctors' visits and drugs. The people believe the advertising which states that the shot "will decrease the effects of the flu should you get it." Which seems like "brain washing" taken to the extreme.

Everything about their marketing is "fear-based", and I have news for you, which is that it works. Here are examples you may have heard:

- if you go outside, you probably need to be screened for skin cancer.

- if you eat fish, you need to be screened for potentially deadly mercury levels.

- if you are over the age of 50, you need to have your colon screened for cancer.

- if you eat meat or dairy, you probably need to have your cholesterol checked and then take medication daily.

I could go on and on, but you can see what they are doing. People hear these advertisements, and it plants the seeds of doubt and fear, which is typically enough to get someone fearful enough to set up appointments for these different potential ailments. Actually, this is what the commercial was meant to accomplish, and that is to get you to spend money on these services.

At the time of this writing, it is 2018 and Health-care Inc. makes up $1/6^{th}$ of the entire economy of the United States. You would think that with all of our technologies and newly advanced therapy break-throughs, we would have hardly any disease. My grand-parents smoked tobacco, drank alcohol, primarily ate eggs, dairy, and meat as their diet. They all lived well into their eighties and were healthy their entire lives until they transitioned. I have friends who live in Ecuador, and they are ex-pats originally from the United States. They have excellent health insurance and their premiums are less than $1/10^{th}$ of what they would pay for much less coverage and much higher deductibles here in the United States. When I learned about how much less expensive it was, and that their healthcare system is excellent, with most of their physicians having been trained in the States, the question begging to be asked was "how does a third-world country do a much better job on healthcare than we do in the United States?" I asked my friend Francisco about it, as he grew up in Ecuador and spent 20 years living in the United States. He said, "The answer is simple, our doctors are not millionaires, and we eat a far healthier diet down here than you do in the States." He brought up another great point, and that was that people in Ecuador eat mostly fresh food that is not processed, and that they drink a lot of fresh juice, which is a large part of their diet as well.

Something is wrong when the price of health care here in the United States costs well over 20X what it does in Ecuador and they are healthier. Our system is based around keeping people sick, as that is where the money is, which is about as flawed as it could possibly be.

Now that we have talked about the money machine that I refer to as Healthcare Inc., let's move on and talk about the true cause of the illusion of ill health.

CHAPTER 2

———

THE TRUE NATURE OF YOUR HUMAN EXPERIENCE

One of the greatest truths ever shared with me is that our entire human experience is just that, an experience. This truth was shared with me by Spirit in January of 2018, and the importance of what I am about to share with you will change not only your world, but also the health and healing for all who come into the human experience now and forever more.

We are all spiritual beings having a human experience. Let me say that again, we are all spiritual beings having a human experience. If you have never heard that before, it might sound a little "out there," but it is not. In my book, *The 7 Master Keys for Success with Deliberate Creation*, I taught about how to consciously create the reality you desire through using my *VisualFestation System*. This was my second book on the subject, which came out seven years after my first book, *VisualFestation*. *VisualFestation* was about the massive success I had with working with the Law of Attraction and manifesting what I desired in my life. This book you are reading will make you question everything that you have ever been told about health and healing. It will also stretch your comprehension about how our realities work in what I like to call "physicality."

We are all here visiting as spirits having a human experience. The experience can best be described as in a dream which you create through your thoughts, beliefs, and feelings. Which is the exact opposite of what the world believes to be true. The world believes that reality is the only thing real, and everything that you experience somehow happens to you through something called "fate". That statement is so wrong for me it is almost incomprehensible. I have proven this to be false through the events I have deliberately created in my own life experience. To deny what I know to be the "truth" after proving it is simply ridiculous. The "truth" about who you are and the power you hold will set you free of any condition, especially with your health.

The same power you have will also cause you to suffer if it is used incorrectly. There is only one "Power," and it is always there working through you and creating your experience based on what you are "thinking in to it." Positive thoughts such as love and gratitude will bring more things in to your life to be grateful for, and equally true is that thoughts based on fear will create a drama or human horror show in your life. If you don't believe me, look at your life until now. Are you happy and healthy, or are you unhappy and sick?

Before you tell yourself that it is something which you had no control over because of _____, I want you to know that's a complete lie because you did. That is the "victim" answer, and it might get you sympathy and attention from others reinforcing that belief, but it is NOT the truth. You had absolutely no idea that you were creating it, as no one has ever shared with you the real truth until now. However, now that you know the truth, it is time to take back your power and create the experience of perfect health and abundance in your life.

This is a decision that only YOU can make, and trust me there will be many people out there who will tell you that what I am sharing with you is wrong. What is wrong is that they have no idea what they are talking about when it comes to how our human experience is created. If they knew, they would be sharing what I know with you instead of disagreeing with the truth. What I am about to tell you IS THE TRUTH, which was shared with me by what I call Spirit, and that is that any diseases are illusions we create and then attach to our experience. They are simply very strong illusions which we have created through the misuse of our thoughts, beliefs, and emotions. The greatest of which is fear.

I like to break out the word "fear" into an acronym with stands for "False Evidence Appearing Real." Which is the perfect definition of what people experience as disease. When you stand back and look at the fearful thoughts you have, you will see that they are all just in your head and not in your reality. Unfortunately, if you keep on having those thoughts, you will have what you fear show up perfectly in your experience and if you are like everyone else on the planet, you probably will believe that you had nothing to do with it. Which is false as you had everything to do with it. Your life and everything in it is one giant self-fulfilling prophecy you create. You are the master of your experience, and it is time for you to accept that responsibility and create the life you desire.

———

CHAPTER 3

THE PARADIGM & ILLUSION

The True Source

The true source of all sickness and disease is thought. Let me explain. Your thoughts, fears, and beliefs either make you sick or they provide you with the experience of perfect health. You may have heard the saying that "thoughts become things". Everything that exists in our human experience is made of energy. There is nothing but energy in our experience, and it appears to be in different forms based on vibration. Your thoughts are energy, and they have their own vibration and they are the source of creation which makes up the individual human experience that you view as your reality. You may need to read that last sentence a few times to truly understand what I am telling you.

What you experience in your reality is created by you; the thoughts you think, and the feelings you have about yourself and your world. If you hold a deep-down fear of a nasty disease and if you keep having thoughts and feelings of fear, you more than likely will have that "disease experience" show up in your reality. It is not punishment from God, it is simply you misusing the creative power of your mind and the appearance of disease in your experience is simply the result of holding those negative thoughts.

Holding and affirming that you are healthy in your thought and being will create and maintain the experience of perfect health. You are always working with natural laws which make up how our experience works. Most people incorrectly believe that life is happening to them and that they have no control over it. Which is one giant myth that most of the world believes to be true. Whatever is happening to you results directly from the thoughts you are thinking. A great analogy is to think of yourself as the writer of the screenplay, the director of the film, and the leading character in the movie called your life. Most people in the world have no idea they are the creators of the experience they live, whether positive or negative.

Once you accept this, you realize that you are 100% responsible for your life and that you can change your outside circumstances through changing your thoughts and beliefs. Another way to think about it is to view your thoughts as though they are the most powerful magnetic force in the universe, and that they are attracting and bringing forth a reality that is a vibration match to your thoughts. Which is essentially the Law of Attraction. The Law of Attraction is a law of our experience always operating in the background bringing forth human experiences that are a match to your dominant thoughts, whether they are feelings of wealth and happiness, or thoughts of poverty, sickness, and sadness. I have written two other books which have proven this Law from my own experience. Our physical reality appears as though it is solid and fixed, but that is just how it appears. It is dynamic and we can change any of it by controlling what we think in to it.

This is good news, as anything that has been created by thought can just as easily be uncreated by thought. You are the miracle healer you have been searching for. But until you radically and completely change what you think and focus on, the healing will be temporarily blocked from your experience. Let me give you an example which I saw through the experience of a close friend of mine. My friend held a deep-down feeling of resentment towards his aunt's family who were wealthy. He and everyone in his family also held the same deep-down feeling it simply wasn't "fair" and felt resentment against their cousins who were born with a "silver spoon in their mouth." Well, after holding on to this resentment and jealousy for over 50 years, my friend had the experience of cancer which ended up killing him in the end. The saddest part of the whole thing was that he didn't even know he was creating it, as the feelings of jealousy and resentment seemed completely normal to him as he had had them his entire life.

The Time is Now

It doesn't matter if you have spent your entire life until now thinking and holding on to negative feelings and emotions such as:

- guilt

- lack of self-love

- hatred

- jealousy

- resentment

- lack of forgiveness

- complaining

- believing you are sickly

It can all change for you right now by removing and replacing those disempowering thoughts with empowering ones. Only you can do this, and your life depends upon it. Accept that you have created everything in your life until now based on ignorance. You probably were never exposed to this truth before, so don't blame or negatively judge yourself. Now that you know this truth there is no reason for you to ever be the "victim" of your thoughts again. Instead, be the victor of your thoughts and create the reality you desire.

The Greatest Secret

The greatest secret that the world is yet to discover is that we are all spiritual beings having a human experience in physicality. We all chose to come here and we have all been here before, and we can return again. One of the ground rules that each of us agreed to was, we had to forget that we were Spirits and that we could create whatever we desired through the proper use of our thoughts and imagination. We all came here for the adventure we know as life and to experience all the things which make up a pleasurable experience such as love, joy, and abundance. Through the misuse of our thoughts and imagination, we create what looks like a "nightmare" in our experience, and that is the illusion of sickness and disease.

The Illusion...

The idea that sickness and disease were illusions we create through thought and the fact that we could remove the experience of suffering through changing our thoughts came directly from Spirit in January of 2018. The information came through intuitive knowing along with a visual experience where the truth was as straightforward as it could be. When the TRUTH comes in, there is no question about it. Believe me. Essentially, the appearance of sickness or disease is an illusion created through thought which we then "attach" to our human experience until we DECIDE TO SHATTER THE ILLUSION THROUGH MASSIVELY CHANGING OUR THOUGHTS, WHICH THEN CHANGE OUR BELIEFS, AND SUBSEQUENTLY, OUR ENTIRE REALITY! Long before I wrote this book of Truth, I knew this would be a hard concept for most of the world to accept and believe at this moment in time.

But then again there is no time like the present to reclaim your perfect health, which is your birthright and which is always available to you when you consciously decide to change your consciousness. I think to describe the process would be to use the term "transformational", as you will be transforming what you are experiencing as your reality and transforming it in to the reality which you desire to experience.

One challenge you will all face is dealing with a paradigm that has been in place since the beginning of time, which is the belief that sickness and disease is something from the outside environment we somehow contract, and that the only way to get rid of it is through outside therapies. That is what most of the world believes to be true, but most of the world is completely WRONG. If you want to keep experiencing more ill health, be like the rest of the world and believe that you are powerless and continue to live in fear. If you want to change your life to one of perfect health, happiness, and abundance, then let's move on to the Seven Steps...

CHAPTER 4

————

STEP ONE: DECIDE

The first step to changing anything and everything is to decide what it is that you say you want. Until you make the formal decision to change what you desire to experience, you are not changing anything, but instead, you are maintaining the status quo of your experience. Perfect health is a choice, and it is and always has been available to you. Your life until now may have looked like the absolute opposite of perfect health. What you have been experiencing until now is still being experienced because you have not yet formally DECIDED to experience perfect health. Deciding to commit to achieving and experiencing perfect health needs to have a lot of powerful "whys" behind it. The major question to ask yourself is, "Why do I REALLY, REALLY, REALLY want to experience perfect health?" The best way I have found to do this is through writing the question on the top of a blank sheet of paper in a notebook, and then to write down the reasons. After each reason that you put down, write out what that would "feel" like to have this decision BE TRUE and manifest into your reality. The importance of having very strong reasons you desire to return to perfect health will keep you focused on doing your part daily until you achieve it.

Another major decision to make is to remove forever any "victim" programs that consciously or unconsciously are running in the background. Let me describe for you an example which I am sure that you have either done yourself or that you have observed in others. One of the things which are universal and true for all of us is that we want to feel love and be loved. Sometimes a way for us to get attention and to feel love from others is through becoming sick. Everyone seeking the feeling of love and attention in this manner continues down this road where each ailment created is worse than the previous one, and if taken to the extremes, you will end up with the illusion of disease which is terminal, incurable, or both. Is this a pattern you have been perpetuating? If it sounds like it could be then it absolutely is. I am not here to pass judgment, I am here to help you uncover negative belief patterns, as you must identify them and stop the process or they will self-sabotage your healing and keep you from experiencing perfect health. Not being honest with yourself and living in denial will not create positive change; instead, it will perpetuate more opportunities for you to feel love as you get sicker and sicker, which is not what you want. Is it?

More Decisions...

One of the major decisions you will need to make is HOW you want to move forward with healing and a return to perfect health. If you are already battling something that you created, you will need to deal with smashing that illusion first. There are a lot of methodologies for treating any "illusion" that we've created, and the most common choices are:

- western medicine and pharmaceuticals

- eastern medicine

- holistic healing

- creative mind and deliberate creation

Or you can mix and match these to find what works best for you. The most important choice you need to make is to choose the one or ones which YOU BELIEVE WILL HEAL YOU. Following a regimen you don't believe will work is a total waste of your time and energy. If you want to see concrete proof about how powerful your mind is, look up the research on drug trials and how well the drugs do compared to the placebos. The placebos are not drugs at all, and in most studies, the placebo has better outcomes with healing people than that actual drug does!

If you want even stronger proof, look at the research of "Second Year Syndrome." Second Year Syndrome refers to what happens to a lot of second-year medical students who study the various types of diseases and then contract the disease just by researching it! When I worked in health care, my boss got some crazy disease as part of Second Year Syndrome, and it made him drop out of med school as he was so sick it almost killed him!! People in medicine see this as just being some crazy phenomenon, but when you understand the real cause of disease, you will see that is EXACTLY WHAT WE ARE TALKING ABOUT, and the medical profession KNOWS this. If you have never heard of Second Year Syndrome before, don't be surprised. It does not usually get out beyond the halls of medicine.

Decide today to heal your life, and it will never look the same again!

_____

CHAPTER 5

STEP TWO: ACTION

Taking back your health involves taking action. Once you take action regularly, the universe will meet you halfway. You are not working and taking action all by yourself, you are working directly with and through Spirit to manifest perfect health. Taking action on both the physical and spiritual planes simultaneously makes everything happen that much quicker for you. We will talk about physical actions first, and then move on to discuss the spiritual work second. Raising your vibration from where it is currently is priority number one, as you must get your body ready to take back its natural strength, and if you have not felt well for a while, it may almost be hard to remember what that is like. It doesn't matter how long it has been, what matters is that you will take action and get back to feeling good again.

The first step to getting your energy on an upward trajectory is to move your body physically. Moving allows the energy inside your body to be just like that of a shark in the ocean. Sharks must keep moving or they drown. The same can be said about your body and physical movement. Where you will start from depends on how long a certain condition has been present in your experience.

It doesn't matter if you find yourself at the moment bedridden, or if you have only recently experienced not feeling well. You MUST TAKE ACTION NOW.

We will discuss visualization further in the chapter, but if you are bedridden at this moment in time, start by closing your eyes and exercise in your mind. Start by seeing yourself getting up out of bed and putting your feet on the floor and then see yourself walking out of your room, then down the corridor and then outside. Do this as often as you can until you are walking by yourself unassisted outside. Once you have done this, you are well on your way back to perfect health. Hopefully, you are at a stage where you can get up and walk on your own. Movement, especially outdoors in nature, can work wonders for your energy. If you must exercise indoors, do that for now, and then increase your energy levels so you can get outside. There is tremendous healing energy for you to tap in to from nature. It could be walking through a beautiful park or garden, or it could be from doing a hike or walking on the beach. There is energy there, and it is there for you to restore you to perfect health. Through exercising and spending time in nature, you will begin to feel better both mentally and physically as your vibration rises as your inner energy.

Besides movement and exercise, another great way for you to raise your vibration physically is to eat better! What and when you eat can have a profound difference on how well you feel. You are trying to increase your vibration and energy, so let's talk about how to do that through what we eat and drink. Most people have diets so bad they only lead to a low vibration and obesity at some level. I lived down South in the United States for almost twenty years, and I have seen first-hand what the long-term effects of eating an unhealthy diet are. In the South, fried food is a big part of the culture and most who have grown up and live there are obese from eating a diet of little more than batter and deep frying. Becoming obese makes it harder and harder for one to exercise, so eventually, you create a body that is extremely overweight, and then it is a lot more difficult to make the changes needed as you have let the process slide for so long.

It doesn't matter where you start from, what is important is taking the actions required and to eat healthier. The first step I suggest, and let me be clear up front, I am not a trained dietician, is to not eat processed foods at all. This will probably require a total change in your eating behavior. Instead of eating macaroni and cheese out of the box for dinner, how about having a salad with light dressing? As soon as you start eating fresh vegetables and fruits, you notice your energy levels are rising and that you are hungry more often as your metabolism is increasing. Rather than eating three large meals a day, graze and eat five smaller meals per day. This again will increase your metabolism. Through increasing your metabolism and exercising, you are going to burn off body fat and lose weight, which again is raising your vibration.

One of the things which seem to have incredible results is to take in large amounts of nutrients from vegetables and plants through what is known as "juicing." I have seen documentaries on people who have made incredible increases in their health through consuming fresh juice which they have made. My wife and I own a juicing machine and you cannot imagine how many nutrients you can extract with a juicer. I can only describe the juice as probably the most vitamin and nutrient food there is. It doesn't make sense to eat a basket of fruit at each sitting, but you can get the equivalent nutrients of that basket in one glass of juice. I cannot recommend juicing fresh fruits and vegetables enough, as they naturally have all the nutrients your body needs, and again it will raise your vibration and make you feel better. Don't take my word for it; look at the research of the beneficial health effects of consuming fresh fruits and vegetables in this manner. It may be just what you have been looking for.

Another simple thing to get your body feeling better and running better is to consume large amounts of fresh water daily. Most of the world lives in some state of dehydration, as they simply do not drink enough water. Drinking things such as alcohol and caffeine dehydrate you even though you are consuming fluids. This is also true about soft drinks, etc. Being hydrated has a wonderful effect on your entire body from your organs to your brain. Being hydrated allows your body to work far more efficiently, and you will notice that you will stop feeling bloated once you drink enough. When you don't take in enough water, your body starts slowing down to protect itself, as it is concerned about when it will be rehydrated again. By drinking water throughout your day, you will keep this protective mechanism in place and keep it from engaging and your body and mind will operate much more efficiently, which is just what we are striving for. Most of you are shaking your heads in agreement to what we just discussed about exercise, healthier eating, and drinking large amounts of water. It is not enough to agree with me, you must commit to doing it every day, and it will change your life and health forever.

Action of the Spiritual Plane

Besides taking action on the physical plane, taking action on the spiritual plane is even more powerful. In short, it is where we connect with all the power in our universe and it concerns tapping into the power of Spirit, the power of God, or what is also known as Christ Consciousness. Whatever you call it, the results are the same, and it is the Power through which we can create miracles in our lives. The Power is always there ready to help, but we must be in alignment for it to work through us to create anything we desire to experience. Describing how this Power works is about as close as I can get to knowing how it works. I don't know how it works, but I know how to work with it and create miracles, and that is precisely what I am about to share with you.

Most people believe that all healing, just like disease, comes from the outside and then is experienced internally as healing or ill health. That is what everyone believes, but it is ABSOLUTELY FALSE. ANYTHING AND EVERYTHING FIRST HAPPENS WITHIN US AS A RESULT OF OUR THOUGHTS AND THEN MATERIALIZES IN TO OUR PHYSICAL REALITY AS A CONDITION OR ILLUSION. Feel free to read that last sentence a few more times to truly get what I am truly conveying to you. Now that you have been exposed to this TRUTH, let me show you how to run the "manifestation machine" you are.

We create our reality. Once you can accept this, you can then change anything and everything in your future including the shattering of the illusion of disease and returning to a state of perfect health, happiness, and abundance. I created what I call my VisualFestation System, which is essentially the technique I have combined and used deliberately to create my human experience. It has gotten me amazing results over the past decade or more, and it will work just as well for you, as we all have the ability to tap in to this Power and create that which we desire.

The next step to creating change in your life experience is to stop buying in to APPEARANCES. What you are seeing in your reality right now, good or bad, results from what you have thought in the past. The past is the past, so don't waste another moment thinking about it. Release the past just like you would a bad-tasting cup of coffee, dump it out, and then walk away from it and never think about it again. Having the result of perfect health begins with you reprogramming your thoughts and beliefs to HEALTH NOW! If you have been thinking horrible thoughts about fear and illness, you must take that same passion and affirm that you have perfect health, and have that become a mantra you say repeatedly throughout your day with the true belief that IT IS SO. Through affirming this as being the truth, it will begin to override the negative thoughts, as there won't be room for them to take root in your garden which now only operates on positivity.

Another technique which I use every day is called Creative Visualization. In my experience, this has been the most powerful technique of all. We are always creating our reality and this technique is like working with dynamite as far as getting results. Scientific research is finally noticing the correlation between visualizing better health and seeing the actual result of better health in the people in the study. They are only scratching the surface on this, as they cannot comprehend what is going on. When you combine visualizing with faith, along with the other VisualFestation techniques, you will demonstrate the fact that this works beyond any shadow of a doubt. To get started, spend a day or two describing in words and then cutting out pictures of what perfect health looks like to you. Take your time with this, as we are all visual people, and having the right picture of what perfect health looks like to us will help us make it easier to visualize. The pictures you select should "speak" to you on a feeling and emotional level. If they don't, stay with the process until you have ones that do. Once you have the pictures, either paste them on a piece of poster board, or put them into a binder. There is no right way or wrong way to do this, so don't worry. Congratulations! You have just created your first vision board or vision book. Now that you have this tool, let me show you how to use it. Find a quiet place where you won't be interrupted for at least twenty minutes by anyone or anything such as an incoming call or text on your phone. Now, look at your pictures and study each one of them to get a feeling of what each one of them represents to you. A picture you may have could be one of a grandparent pushing a child on a swing and they both are smiling. That represents you being active, healthy, and feeling the love of spending time with your grandchildren. That feeling of love is powerful and is just what we are after.

After reviewing the pictures, relax and close your eyes, and see yourself in your "mind's eye" having the experience of living your life as if everything on the board was true. This is not to be confused with day-dreaming; this is a powerful and deliberate use of creative visualization where you are combining emotions to the things you are visualizing. When you are ready to complete the visualization exercise, see everything you have visualized contained in a giant pink bubble, and see that everything has a pink hue to it. Then, see this balloon rise to the heavens and eventually disappear. Now open your eyes, and know that you have done your part, and that God or Spirit will take care of making it happen for you. I practice creative visualization every single morning, and feel free to do the same exercise while you lie in bed before you go to sleep for best results. When you have done this technique properly, you will have tears of joy in your eyes when you come out of the exercise, as that is just how powerful this technique is.

Another technique which I practice is called Scripting, and it is almost like you are writing down on paper, with feeling, what you would be visualizing. One of the most important things you need to do is to make what you script about be what YOU DE-SIRE, and not what anyone else wants. THIS IS ALL ABOUT YOU. PERIOD! I keep a journal just for scripting, and I always put the date on the top of the page. I do this because I like to look back on what I have scripted in the past and when I wrote it, and then to see how long it took to manifest in to my current reality. The life I am living today was something I first scripted and visualized first in my mind and it has become my reality. The same will BE TRUE FOR YOU.

Let's assume again that you are a grandparent and that you may be experiencing the illusion of disease. Here's what a scripting session might look like to you. "Lord I cannot THANK YOU ENOUGH FOR MY TOTAL AND COMPLETE HEALING!!! I feel wonderful and I don't think that I have ever felt better! Everyone is telling me about how amazing I look, and they all want to know my secret about looking so healthy and beautiful at my age! The best part of feeling great is all the energy I have and all the fun I have playing with the grandkids. I know someday they will grow up so I am not missing a second to play with them and teach them how to make chocolate chip cookies which we all love and enjoy. I cannot express the joy and love I feel and for the time I have with them and for my COMPLETE HEALING!

THANK YOU LORD BEYOND WORDS!"

I don't have grandchildren, but I can honestly say that it brought in the feeling of raw love and emotion as I wrote it. When you can script that which you desire and combine it with massive positive emotion, you will have this technique down and I suggest you do it every single day.

Another powerful technique that I use is one I call "As If...", where I think, speak, and act as if my miracle has already come true and I am living it in the moment. It is an easy technique to practice, but do not think for a moment that it is not powerful, because it is. *As an example: Imagine yourself getting a call from your doctor's office, and the only thing they can say is that they have just witnessed a MIRACLE and that the disease is gone!* Now act as though that was true and just happened. What would you be saying to God? Don't think it, SAY IT! Get into a feeling of total gratitude like you cannot imagine, and stay with it as long as you can and KNOW that the phone call telling you the same is on its way to you, and again give THANKS!

Combining the ACTIONS of both the physical world along with the spiritual world will produce health and healing to you in a way that will amaze everyone around you. They will be the witnesses of something that they never believed could be true and that is you manifesting perfect health!

Now let's move on to the next step and which is focus.

CHAPTER 6

STEP THREE: FOCUS

A crucial step to reclaiming your perfect health is through developing your ability to maintain absolute focus on that which you desire. Most people in the world are spending all of their time focusing on what they don't want and they don't even realize they are doing it. If you called them on it, they would undoubtedly say it is just "normal" and "of course, I am focused on it, wouldn't you be if you had my life?" What the world does not realize, however, is that whatever you focus your thoughts and attention to brings more and more of it into your experience. It is simply just another example of the Law of Attraction in action, and it is always working and bringing more of what you are thinking about and focusing on back to you.

Focusing your thoughts and energy on sickness and disease will bring you the experience of more sickness and disease. We live in a thought-driven experience, so understand it, know it, and use it to create perfect health and healing instead of the appearance of sickness in to your experience. I know there are many people who after reading that will say, "That's easy for you to say, as you don't have _____ disease." If that is what you are thinking, you will need to drop it, as that is 100% pure "victim speak," and it is a very clear example of what you need to be working on. Developing the ability and mastery of focus whereby you focus on only that which you desire regardless of appearances in your reality is a powerful skill for manifesting. Most people will tell you they are focused, but when something challenging shows up, they immediately start focusing on the challenge. They give it more energy instead of the opposite, which is an inner peace from knowing that everything is working out perfectly and a complete healing is on its way. Mastering the skill of focus is something that more than likely will take time, as you have been using that skill for all the wrong reasons for most of your life. To master the skill of focus, you will need to pay attention to your thoughts. Once you do that, you will be overwhelmed at the percentage of negative thoughts you think compared to the number of positive and empowering thoughts you think daily. Nothing is wrong with you, that is exactly how the rest of the world thinks too! But we are striving to return to perfect health; therefore, we must do the exact opposite if we desire to get better results.

Maintaining your focus on complete healing and perfect health is truly a life or death mission you are on in your experience. Through the misuse of focus, you will get sicker or worse; through the proper use of focus, you will rise and reclaim your perfect health. Out of all the circumstances we may find ourselves in, the ability to focus on health within your mind and to stay with it while on the outside the appearance of a negative health tsunami is happening, is powerful beyond words.

You too are powerful beyond words; you may have temporarily forgotten that fact. Here are key points I need to share with you that will help you realize the power of focus:

1. We are all living in a thought-based and thought-creative human experience. Everything that you see on the outside is being created by you on the inside. If you will change what you focus on internally with your mind, you will change what you experience externally as your reality.

2. Everything you see in your outer experience CAN BE CHANGED BY YOU. ALL OF IT. But it will require you to stop focusing on appearances and instead for you to focus on that which you desire and bring it forth from the unseen to the seen.

The time is now for you to completely and unequivocally focus on a complete healing and perfect health. I

KNOW THAT YOU CAN DO THIS, SO DON'T WASTE ANOTHER DAY. Commit right now to focusing only on healing and let the illusion of disease wither away and disappear from your experience forever.

CHAPTER 7

————

STEP FOUR: FAITH

Having true and undeniable faith that you are creating perfect health and shattering the illusion of disease is about as powerful as anything in our entire universe. Unfortunately, most people in our world relate the word "faith" with religion. Most religions preach a gospel that essentially says, "Do what we tell you and you will get to heaven. Don't do what we tell you and you will pay the consequences for eternity." That is ignorance of how Spirit works and it is man's way of exercising control over people and their wallets. When I refer to faith, I am referring to faith in a God/Spirit and faith in ourselves and our ability to co-create that which we desire.

Adequately describing and conveying what faith is when it comes to successfully manifesting miracles is a deep topic as most people's level of faith is somewhere along the lines of "hope." Having a level of faith best described by the level of hope, is almost like having no faith whatsoever! It is so weak that you may as well not even bother. That might sound harsh, but that is the truth.

One of the greatest challenges most people have when they create and experience the illusion of disease is to somehow believe either that God has abandoned them or somehow there is a lesson to be learned and it is God's will that they are sick. If that is what you believe right now, you are going to need to drop these false beliefs now and forever more. God wishes only joy and happiness for all of us, all the time! We create these false appearances and then experience them in our reality. The great news is that through working in faith, we can create anything that we desire to experience.

I think the best way to describe the level of faith that I am referring to would be to describe it as a deep-down "knowing," where it is not really something just in your mind, but it is truly a part of your being. Taking it even to a higher level is when you KNOW THAT IT IS DONE. At this level, we have dropped all "ifs", and now it is just WHEN. This is the level we all need to be at to maximize our co-creator powers and most efficiently manifest our desired reality.

When your faith temporarily slides, and you have the fear-based thoughts of doubt and think something along the lines of "what if it doesn't work?", you are creating roadblocks and delays to your complete healing taking place in your experience. Have utter and undeniable faith in your ability to manifest miracles through Spirit and IT SHALL BE.

―――――

CHAPTER 8

STEP FIVE: CONSISTENCY

One thing which I am most noted for is my practice of what I call my "hour of power," and the fact that I have not missed doing it a single day since I began doing it over fifteen years ago. A major factor in my success with manifesting is my consistency. I wake up every morning and practice the techniques of my VisualFestation System. It doesn't matter if I am at home or on the road, I bring everything that I need with me when I travel as I know how important consistency is to manifesting.

Shattering the illusion of disease will take a massive commitment. You must commit to doing your part every single day until perfect health is again your reality. When I refer to your part, I am referring to doing all the exercises in the step called action. Reading and thinking about it will not give you the results you desire. Your life and making positive changes to it is anything but a spectator sport. Instead, imagine that you are a gladiator and the only way to gain your freedom is through slaying the illusion of disease. If you don't give everything you have to winning this battle, you may not get another chance to compete in the arena. When you look at it in that manner, I am sure that you are saying, "I am ready! Let's go!"

One of the most common questions that most people ask is "How long is it going to take me to return to perfect health?" That is a great question and I wish I knew the answer. The entire process of reclaiming your perfect health comes down to you. Only you know what you are thinking about or are fearing, and how long it will take for each one of us will be different. The process ALWAYS WORKS and you are working with Spirit, so don't think for a second there is anything that God cannot do through you. Being consistent on your part will make things happen for you that much sooner.

Commit to doing your hour of power every single morning when you get up and do nothing else until you have completed it. Also, do all the other action items every day as well. Drink plenty of water, eat better, and get outside and move. The greatest athletes in the world never skip practice, and if you want over-the-top results, you won't either! You are playing a game with stakes so high you cannot afford to give it anything but all that you have. I know there are some people reading this and saying something like, "I don't have time to do my hour of power because of _____." If you are not willing to do your part on a consistent and daily basis, you simply do not want to be healed enough, because if you did there would be nothing you wouldn't do to return to perfect health. Working with Spirit or God, whichever you prefer is NOT something that you dabble in occasionally. Dabbling will not get you results, consistency will. Your perfect healing is waiting on you, but you must show up every day like your life depends on it because it DOES!

CHAPTER 9

STEP SIX: AWARENESS

The next step we will discuss is awareness. The concept of awareness is deep, and it is becoming aware of the energies around you and how they are shaping your thoughts and influencing your human experience. Negativity is everywhere, so be on the watch for these influences and identify them for what they are, which is negative, that way you can consciously decide to move away from them. More than likely, you have people in your life, whether they be friends, family, or co-workers, who are negative or worse yet, "toxic." What I am about to say may sound "harsh", but you get anyone who is negative out of your life. It doesn't matter if they have been a friend of yours for years or not. Negative people sap your inner energy and lower your vibration. For healing, we need to get your vibration high and keep it there.

Once you observe and become more aware, you will notice that almost everything that you see, read, or hear is 99% negative. A great example of this is called "the news." "The news" is simply bad news, and listening to a bunch of tragic events all over the world does not make you informed, it just lowers your vibration. The worse the news is, the greater the listenership, which equates to higher advertising revenue. I don't know why most people like to hear about how bad the world is and how it is getting worse every second. Do yourself a favor and turn it off. You have bigger fish to fry than hearing about a crisis 10,000 miles away that has nothing to do with you or your healing.

One of the greatest things you must be aware of is how you are self-identifying with your experience with the illusion of disease. Most people view themselves as "victims" of disease, and then they spend all of their time talking with others who have experienced the same illusion. To make matters even worse from an awareness standpoint, is when the illusion of disease in your experience becomes who you are or you allow the disease to become who you are. When you self-identify as the disease or the face of the disease, all you are doing is giving more attention to it, which is only making it more powerful in your experience. If this is what you are doing, you need to become aware of the fact that you are "aiding and abetting" the enemy!

I have met people who have literally had the illusion of eight forms of a single disease, and I know it will not stop there, as the only conversation and thought they think is about the disease and what is going on with it yesterday, today, and tomorrow. If that sounds anything like you, you must get honest about what you are doing to yourself.

Another topic I need to discuss with you is the support and larger so-called disease awareness organizations. For anyone who understands the true nature of our experience, these groups are simply creating more and more of the disease as people become afraid of it, and subsequently, they create the illusion in their reality. If you want to experience more disease, keep going to rallies and marches where the attention is focused on disease.

On a much smaller scale, but one just as powerful, is what you are telling yourself about the likelihood of a potential disease? Are you calling it forth in to your experience by thinking things such as:

> "_____ disease runs in our family."
> "My grandmother and mother both had it, so it is just a matter of time before I get it."

Your words and thoughts create your reality so be aware of what you are saying and thinking every single moment of the day.

Another part of being aware which is more pleasant to talk about is, you are not here alone and you have spiritual helpers always available to you. I didn't quite understand this either until around three years ago. After deep meditations, I became aware that I have always had spirit guides and guardian angels with me my entire life. Looking back on my life and seeing crazy things happen for me, like not getting killed on my motorcycle or in a crazy car accident, it was obvious that I had help from the unseen which appeared to be just some crazy good luck! After doing the meditations and being reminded of all the times they intervened in to my experience to keep me safe was amazing. I know this might sound too "out there" for you at this time, trust me, I get it, but I want you to know that you always have help available to you for anything and everything, so don't feel as though you must go it alone. Nothing is "cool" about suffering when you can make the choice not to. Your guides and angels have a number of different ways in which to communicate with you. The first step though is that you must acknowledge them and want to meet and work with them to help heal you. I have been working with my spirit guides for three short years, and I am now at the level where I can ask a question and get a very clear answer back. This is helpful, especially when things on the surface of my reality resemble pure chaos. If you want to learn more about communicating with your angels and spirit guides, I suggest reading some of the works produced by Doreen Virtue or Gil Alan.

Live an aware life starting from today and remove any negativity from your life. If you do so, you will find that the road back to perfect health will be much shorter than you ever imagined!

CHAPTER 10

STEP SEVEN: GRATITUDE

The seventh step to reclaiming perfect health is gratitude. The only emotion stronger than gratitude is love, which is the most powerful force in our universe. One of the most important things you must do if you want to achieve amazing results is to practice gratitude right now. Right now, you have plenty to be grateful for. If you are reading this book, you are alive and that is something to be grateful for. There are way too many things that most of us take for granted which we shouldn't as things could change and the blessings you take for granted could go away. To put things in perspective, how important is having eye-sight and the ability to see to you? Important, I am sure you would say. OK then, when was the last time you thanked God for your ability to see? It is so easy to build a long list of blessings you have in your life even if you are temporarily experiencing the illusion of ill health.

Here are more important blessings that almost all of us have, and we must recognize how important these things are in our lives and have gratitude for them now. Besides the importance of seeing, what about your ability to walk? Do you know how much of an incredible challenge every minute of your life would be if you were confined to a wheelchair or bed? How about having all your limbs? How much more challenging would your life be if you had no arms? I could go on and on listing all these wonderful blessings you have in your life which you more than likely have been taking for granted your entire life, unless you have lost them.

Did you have food today and a warm bed to sleep in last night? If you did, do you know what it would be like to not have these blessings? We all have many things to be grateful for in our lives, but unfortunately, most people focus on what they don't have. Through focusing on and feeling frustrated about what you don't have, you are only "crowding out" space for feeling gratitude. The easiest thing that any of us can do to make our lives better is to have GRATITUDE NOW! You already have a huge laundry list of things to be grateful for, so give thanks now. Once you put out the vibration of gratitude, things will change in a positive way in your life. I cannot tell you adequately in words how magnificently powerful having gratitude is or how it can transform your entire reality. One of the greatest secrets to manifesting that I have discovered and practiced successfully in my own life, is having GRATITUDE NOW FOR ALL THE THINGS THAT ARE ON THEIR WAY TO ME. Saying thank you beforehand seems to have this magical way of having it appearing in your experience that much sooner. That is why it is so important for you to have GRATITUDE NOW for your perfect health and healing. Knowing it is done and on its way to you and all the while having gratitude for it now is more powerful than you could imagine.

If there was only one thing I could share with you about successfully manifesting anything in your life, it would be the importance of having gratitude in all areas of your life. When you say thank you to God, you get more things to be grateful for in your life and the process continues constantly as long as you stay in the vibration of gratitude. If you have ever wondered how awesome your life could be, simply stay in gratitude and hold on to your hat as it is going to be an amazing ride to a life that is more beautiful than you can imagine, and it is there waiting for you right now.

Miracles

Miraculous and spontaneous healing takes place every day around the world. You just never hear about it happening, as it is usually done in the privacy of a home or hospital, and it is never heard about by anyone except close friends and family members of those who have manifested healing in such a way. I think we would see countless more examples than we do right now if people understood that disease is an illusion. Through understanding it is an illusion that each of us has created, it makes it that much easier to take charge of our thoughts and beliefs and shatter the illusion.

To give you a concrete example of this, let me share with you an amazing story shared with me by a person who had a total and miraculous healing, and who later became a student of mine. Before I get to the healing part, let me describe what my student's life was like up until this time. As a child, my student had been abused sexually by someone in her family. Having been abused left her with a lot of guilt, and she struggled with self-confidence, and a feeling of "how could a loving God allow such a thing to happen to an innocent child?" These thoughts and feelings stayed with her every day of her life, and they were so powerful that by the time she was in her early thirties, she had been diagnosed with a deadly disease and she was given weeks to live. As part of her end-of-life care, she was placed in hospice, where the staff tried to make her as comfortable as they could while they waited for her to transition, or so they thought!

My student told me the story directly as a first-hand account. She said that she was in hospice and that the doctors and staff all thought she was about to die. She told me that something came over her and filled her with the message to "get out of bed, you are no longer sick." In that moment, she knew that it was the TRUTH and that she was healed. She got out of bed and told the staff she was healed and that she had to get out of hospice as there was no reason for her to be there anymore. The staff thought she had lost her mind and they did everything to convince her she was about to die and to get back in bed. She had to fight with the staff to get released from the hospice facility. Shortly after being released she saw her doctor, who had been overseeing her care, and the doctor could not believe that he could find no trace of the disease in her body, and it was as if it had never even happened.

My student was very open and candid with me, and she knew that the tragic events of the abuse and how she carried it throughout her life were the actual source of the illusion of disease which had manifested into her experience. She really could not explain the healing part except that it was almost like her inner spirit was yelling at her, "What the hell are you doing? I can't take this anymore! Let's get out of here!" After being healed and leaving hospice, she realized that she had to spend time in communion with Spirit and forgive the person who abused her so she could move on and release all the negative energy which had been with her for many years. She did this and it was like taking the weight of the world off her shoulders.

Her story which she has shared with many other people is fascinating, especially as she relayed how her life and health kept getting progressively worse as she stayed in this orbit of guilt and hatred, which eventually led her to being in hospice. She is very grateful to have her health back and she has lost an incredible amount of body fat which she put on over several years of inactivity. To see her before and after pictures was amazing, and her story of healing to this day is something that I share with as many people as I can.

Realize, that you don't have to wait until you get to where you are at death's door to have a miraculous healing. It can happen in a moment and that moment is now. Please do not spend any more time living in the illusion of disease, when you do not have to. Your healing is up to you, so take charge and make it happen by letting God work through you to return you to a state of perfect health which is there and waiting for you.

I pray from the bottom of my heart that the words in this book have touched something inside of you and reminded you of your true greatness. Remember that we are all spirits having a human experience, and the illusion of disease is just an illusion we create. Let me ask each of you a deep and powerful question: "How can a spiritual being ever be sick...YOU'RE RIGHT, IT CAN'T, AND THAT IS THE TRUTH OF YOUR EXPERIENCE!

I wish you Godspeed on your return to your true reality of perfect health.

All the Best,

Pete

APPENDIX

To make it easier for you to create your system and return to perfect health, I have enclosed my *VisualFestation Guide to Healing* below. Just to let you know how powerful this guidebook is, let me share with you the story about how it came about. Around five years ago, I was approached by an older woman who had heard me speak and had read my book, *VisualFestation*. She approached me after a talk I gave and she asked me if there was anything that I could do to help her granddaughter. She then went on to tell me that her eight-year-old granddaughter, Sandy, had just been diagnosed with leukemia and she asked me if there was anything that I could do in any way to help them heal her.

I was having a hard time comprehending that this woman had enough faith in me to help heal her grand-daughter. I agreed to help her on the spot, and I told her I had been contemplating doing something with health and healing, but until then it had just been an idea. Knowing the extreme importance of help-ing a friend save a child's life, I created the eBook on healing, and I sent it to Sandy's grandmother who thanked me graciously. She told me that the book had come at a crucial time as Sandy had just received a bone marrow transplant, and that she had given the book to her daughter who was familiar with my work. A little over a year went by when I came across the grandmother's email address in a stack of business cards in my desk. I remembered that she was Sandy's grandmother, so I sent her an email to ask how Sandy was doing. She emailed me back and told me that Sandy had made a complete recovery and that she was heading back to school in the fall. I cannot tell you how amazing it was to hear that news, and it brought tears of joy to my eyes as I read the note. If you will take the information you are about to learn and run with it, there is nothing that you cannot overcome. Trust me, this stuff works!

The VisualFestation
Guide to Healing

A Law of Attraction Guide to Return You to
Perfect Health

By

Peter D. Adams

Dedication

This book is dedicated to Sandy.

Table of Contents

INTRODUCTION

This book was written especially for you. If you have found this book, it is not by accident. This book was created to give you all the tools you will need to manifest a complete healing. There is nothing you cannot be, do, or have on this planet if you believe you can.

If that sounds a little hard to believe, then you should read my first book entitled, *VisualFestation: How I Manifested the Life of My Dreams & YOU CAN TOO*! In that book, I share with the reader the miracles I have manifested, and the techniques I used which make up the **Visual***Festation* **System**. We now have students from all over the world practicing our *System* and manifesting miracles in their own lives.

I look forward to hearing about your personal success, as I know if you do the work, you will get the results you're looking for.

Godspeed to you.

Pete

LESSON ONE
You HAVE the POWER

There is truly nothing you cannot BE, DO, or HAVE in this world, and that includes enjoying PERFECT HEALTH. You may have been diagnosed as having some horrible disease. However, the most important thing for you to realize is that diagnosis is something in your PAST.

The past has no power except for what we CHOOSE to believe about it, so let's commit to BE-ING IN THE NOW and creating our future. Here, a future that involves a complete healing and the enjoyment of perfect health.

We all can create miracles in our lives. I am going to say it again, **WE ALL HAVE THE ABILITY TO CREATE MIRACLES IN OUR LIVES!** You are more powerful than you can imagine. Your power comes from within, and it has been given to you by God.

You are a Co-Creator in your life, and you have created your life by the thoughts, feelings, and beliefs you have thought or held. Whether you choose to believe this or not, either way, it is true. Through understanding this principle and applying it in our lives, we CAN CREATE MIRACLES IN OUR LIVES AND CHANGE OUR FUTURE.

When I first heard these principles myself, I too found them hard to believe, as it went against everything I had ever been taught before. When I created what later became known as my "12 Crazy Goals," I honestly figured that I had nothing to lose, so why not see if this "stuff" worked. Well, it WORKED, I MEAN IT REALLY WORKED!!! It worked so well that I wrote an entire book about it, and I continue to MANIFEST MIRACLES IN MY LIFE BY PRACTICING THESE TECHNIQUES WHICH I WILL SHARE WITH YOU LATER IN THIS BOOK.

What I have realized is that we were taught how to do this by Jesus over two thousand years ago. I will share with you a few short verses from the New Testament where Jesus essentially describes the whole process on how to manifest miracles.

"ASK AND IT IS GIVEN"

"Ask and it will be given you: seek and ye shall find: knock and it shall be opened unto you: For everyone that asketh receiveth: and he that seeketh findeth: and to him who knocketh it shall be opened."

(Mathew 7:7-8)

"For verily I say unto you, That whosoever shall say unto this mountain, Be thou removed, and be thou cast in to the sea: and shall not doubt in his heart, but shall believe those things which he saith shall come to pass: he shall have whatsoever he saith. Therefore I say unto you, What things soever ye desire when ye pray, believe that ye receive them, and ye shall have them."

(Mark 11:23-24)

"Neither shall they say, Lo here! or, lo there! for, behold, the kingdom of God is within you."

(Luke 17:21)

In the verses above, Jesus, in no uncertain terms is telling us:

Ask for whatever it is that we want.

There is nothing we cannot have if we believe we can have it.

And lastly, that we have the power of God within each and every one one of us.

The whole creation process boils down to ASK, BE-LIEVE, and RECEIVE. You are asking to be healed, and with faith *IT WILL BE SO*. **THAT IS THE ABSOLUTE** *TRUTH*.

I will close this chapter out with this affirmation:

"I AM HEALED. LORD, I CANNOT THANK YOU ENOUGH!!!"

Say this affirmation repeatedly throughout the day and get in to the feeling of gratitude for it being TRUE and that IT IS ON ITS WAY TO YOU!

LESSON TWO

The Power of Forgiveness

Many people suffer from an ailment as adults, which is the result of carrying around toxic "feelings" about an event or a person from the past that hurt you. Sometimes we are not even aware that we hold feelings still, as we may have buried them deep within ourselves and we just don't "go there."

Whether we "go there" or not, that negative energy is still there and present within us. One way to get rid of this energy is through forgiveness. Sometimes people believe that through holding on to re-

sentment they are somehow harming the "offender."
Unfortunately, when one does, this they play the role
of being the "victim." There is no power in playing
the "victim." There *is* power though from forgiving.

Forgiving others gets rid of the "toxic" energy
within us, and the same goes for forgiving ourselves
for anything that we have been beating up ourselves
about. Forgive yourself, forgive them, and release that
energy so you can raise your healing vibration. You
are doing this for you, not for them.

A great exercise for forgiveness is to put the name
of the person on the top of a blank piece of paper, and
then right down all the bad feelings you have been
holding on to from them and the past. When you
finish writing down all these negative feelings on the
paper, go outside and safely set fire to it. Let the paper

burn and feel the energy from those negative energies being released from you, then give thanks they are no longer part of your experience. Remember the principle that to forgive is divine.

Affirm:

"I AM HEALED. LORD, I CANNOT THANK YOU ENOUGH!!!"

LESSON THREE
Medicine & Healing

There have been numerous studies done which have attempted to explain the "placebo effect." Scientists are often baffled when testing an actual drug on one group of people with an ailment while giving sugar pills to a control group of people also suffering from the same ailment. Often, more people in the control group given the placebo drug receive an improvement to their condition equally as well if not better than the group who got the real drug.

Both groups BELIEVED they were getting the

actual drug, which proves that the mere BELIEF that the drug works is as strong as the actual medicine. This proves that the mind can easily create the same outcome as the medicine.

Until recently, big pharmaceutical companies were barred from advertising their drugs on television and radio by the Federal Government. There was a reason for this, and it was because of the power of suggestion.

The research showed that the mere suggestion of symptoms can be enough to convince a person that they have a condition, which then manifests into the actual disease within that person. Your beliefs can easily make you sick, just as easily as they can make you well. If as many people are getting healed from the placebo as the actual drug, can you imagine how powerful you are when you work with the spiritual laws of the universe? In a word, you are **UNSTOPPABLE! BELIEVE IT!**

Through working with and through God, which is what you are doing with Visual*Festation*, **NO MIRACLE IS OUT OF REACH FOR YOU!**

Affirm:

"I AM HEALED. LORD, I CANNOT THANK YOU ENOUGH!!!"

LESSON FOUR
Quantum Physics & Energy

Quantum physics is a very complicated subject, and I cannot say that I am an expert on the topic. Rather than make this a technical discussion on quantum theory, I prefer to simplify it for you.

Everything in our universe when broken down into the smallest building blocks is one thing, and that is energy. Everything you see, feel, taste, etc., is composed entirely of energy. You may never have thought of this before, but you are also comprised of energy. If you looked at your body through a powerful microscope, you would see that at the smallest level, you are energy.

To take it one step further, your spirit or soul, whichever feels more comfortable to you, is also energy. In this case, it is Divine energy.

Is It a "Wave" or a "Particle"?

Quantum physics is the study of subatomic particles, the smallest building blocks of matter, and how they react. One of the most fascinating things that scientists discovered is that when they measured subatomic "particles," depending on the test performed, the result was that the particle could be a "particle" or a "wave." It was probability amplitude, whereby it was simultaneously both a particle and a wave. If that wasn't strange enough, they then did further experiments and concluded the "observer" affected the outcome of the experiment just through observation.

The amazing thing this proved was that the researchers' thoughts were affecting the outcome of the experiments. Thoughts were real things with the energy to shape the outcome. What this told us was that the entire universe is made of this "energy," and that outcomes could be manipulated by our thoughts.

At this energy level we are connected to Source Energy, which is also the level of creation in the universe. This is where your healing will come from.

Affirm:

"I AM HEALED. LORD, I CANNOT THANK YOU ENOUGH!!!"

LESSON FIVE
Purposeful Thought

Now that you know your thoughts affect the outcomes in your physical experience, I cannot over-stress the importance of effectively managing what you think about. Being energy and having a measurable vibration, the thoughts you think on a continual basis, whether good or bad, will attract in events and experiences of a similar vibration.

The simplest way I can describe this to you is through this analogy. Imagine The universe is a giant mail order catalog, and the way that you place your order is through the thoughts you think. On the other end, imagine there is a shipping clerk, the clerk has no idea that size 8 is not what you wanted, because, being diligent, he is just filling the order as requested, so you get a size 8 in your life! If you want a size 4 to show up, order and focus on getting the size 4, not on the size 8.

The power in the truth of the above analogy is immense, and it will change your life once it is understood, and purposeful thought is practiced ongoing.

Whenever thoughts of fear show up, mentally show them the door and tell them they are no longer welcome. It takes vigilance, especially when things don't appear to go your way. You can control what you think about, so commit to purging negative fear-based thinking from your life. You will immediately feel better once you do.

Now that we have gotten rid of those "wrong" thoughts, it is time to replace them with the "right" thoughts. One of the most important "right" thoughts you can think is to focus on gratitude for the things in your life and for the blessings now on their way to you. You may be thinking, "How can I feel gratitude for something that I don't yet have?" Let me give you one of the greatest keys to the Kingdom of Heaven. The sooner you practice gratitude and faith for the blessings you have now, and for those which are on their way, the sooner they will manifest into your experience.

Gratitude is really love, and that is by far the most powerful vibration in the universe. If there is anything you want to be thinking, projecting, and attracting, it is LOVE! Creating the life of your dreams comes down to the quality of your thoughts and having real gratitude for your life now for what you have and that which IS on its way to you!

Have gratitude now for the job of your COMPLETE HEALING, as you will be attracting it in soon based on Natural Law.

Affirm:

"I AM HEALED. LORD, I CANNOT THANK YOU ENOUGH!!!"

LESSON SIX
Feelings Powerful

You may think that I misnamed this chapter, and think that "Powerful Feelings," or "Feeling Powerful" would have "sounded" better. Your feelings have immense energy and power, and they act as nature's warning signs regarding the thoughts you are thinking and thereby attracting. Negative thoughts will make you physically sick, or worse if you continue to think them. That is why when you entertain scary thoughts, you sometimes become nauseous and feel sick to your stomach, or that you immediately come down with a bad headache.

Your body is telling you in a voice as loud as it can to say stop thinking like this, as it knows better and it is trying to get you back on track. Good thoughts feel good, bad thoughts feel bad. Knowing how powerful our feelings are, we can harness this power to work for us through simply changing what we are focusing on and feeling about.

Focus on your HEALING, and then get into the feeling of how good it will feel when it gets here and get into the knowing it is already done. When you align your thoughts and feelings with faith that "IT IS" truly on its way to you, you will become UN-STOPPABLE!

Affirm:

I AM HEALED. LORD, I CANNOT THANK YOU ENOUGH!!!"

LESSON SEVEN
You ARE a Co-Creator of Your Experience

There have been numerous books (this one included), and recently, a movie, all about the Law of Attraction and the process of creation. I know we discussed this in Chapter One, but it is SO important that I am discussing it again so that you REALLY get it.

"Ask, believe, and receive" was told to us nearly two thousand years ago by Jesus and was recorded in the Bible in the book of Mathew 7: 7-8:

"Ask and it shall be given you; seek and ye shall find; knock, and it shall opened unto you: For every

one that asketh receiveth; and he that seeketh find-
eth; and to him that knocketh it shall be opened."

A question you may want to ask yourself is, "Why, after all this time, do we still not 'get it?'" A lot of people have been told by various religions that somehow "God" is separate from them, that they are not worthy, and if they don't follow their dogma, they are going to spend the rest of their days in a hot place, and they don't call it Florida.

Nothing could be further from the truth. There is a piece of the "Creator" inside you, and you have the power to create miracles in your life. I wrote my first book ***VisualFestation*** *How I Manifested the Life of My Dreams and You Can TOO!* to convey that message to you and to share the techniques I have used successfully to create the miracles in my life.

One thing most books fail to get across is that you MUST TAKE ACTION. I define this as the "Co-Creator" piece. In your role as "Co-Creator," there are several job duties that come with the position:

- Decide what you want, why you want it, and focus on your desire for it.

- Believe that you have the power within you to create anything!

- Get into the "feeling" of already having it.

- Have gratitude and believe that it is already on its way to you.

- Avoid anyone who says that you cannot be, do, or have the object of your desire.

- Practice the techniques in this book daily until you receive what you desire.

- If you need a skill to do whatever you say you want, you must take specific action to acquire that skill.

- Permanently commit to removing procrastination from your life.

- Stay out of the "hows" and leave that job up to the universe. The universe reorders itself to make your miracles come true, you need not know "how."

- Develop the skill of endurance, as this is a life-long journey, and sometimes, you may doubt that everything is working.

If you fulfill your duties as "Co-Creator," you will have whatever you say you want. The universe will see to it.

Affirm:

"I AM HEALED. LORD, I CANNOT THANK YOU ENOUGH!!!"

LESSON EIGHT

VisualFestation System Technique: Creative Visualization, Vision Books & Boards

If you have read or listened to my first book, *VisualFestation* or have heard me being interviewed on The Law of Attraction Radio Network, you already know the amazing success I have experienced through using these techniques. One of the most powerful things I do is what I call my **"Hour of Power."** This is the time I use daily to practice The **Visual***Festation* **System** in my own life, and for me, the best time is first thing in the morning.

One of my favorite and most practiced techniques is called Creative Visualization, and the power of this technique, when done properly, will manifest miracles in your life as well.

Seeing how this is a guide for healing, we will tailor the techniques to attracting in a complete healing and a return to perfect and abundant health.

To begin, we will create either a vision book or board, or as I do, both. If this is your first exposure to the concept of vision boards, they are simply visual representations of what your ideal scene would look like. Through the use of pictures that are cut out from magazines or pictures from websites which are then pasted on a lightweight foam board. These can also be created on your computer. The most important thing is to find the best pictures you can to represent the scenes of your desired life. Then, put yourself in those images and scenes, and know that it will happen.

I would suggest cutting out pictures of people smiling and living an active lifestyle. Depending on your current age, you could cut out pictures of people your age spending time with their friends and family. These pictures all must show people smiling and being happy.

To make it real, I would suggest having a friend take a picture of you holding a small sign that says something like, "100% Healed", and maybe another one where you are holding another sign saying, "I Have Perfect Health" and place them on your board.

Keep the board where you can see it frequently to remind yourself of your healing. The boards are used to assist you with creating a visual picture in your mind's eye as to what your reality will look like with complete healing.

Creative Visualization is a technique which I have used with amazing success. When I practice Creative Visualization, I am doing three things simultaneously. I am running a movie in my head where I am visualizing what I want as already being done and in my experience, while simultaneously having a feeling of tremendous joy and gratitude it is TRUE, and giving thanks to the universe for it being SO.

To begin, I find a quiet place to meditate which is free from distractions. I then position myself seated upright with my back straight, and then I inhale and exhale deeply three times with my eyes open. I then shut my eyes and begin to give thanks to the universe for all that I am grateful for, while seeing it visually in my mind's eye. For this example, I would include thanking the universe for giving me a complete healing. I would then see and feel a beautiful beam of a healing, magnificent, white light coming down from the heavens and reaching me. I would then see it gradually and slowly moving down from my head to my feet, and I would know this is the healing light of God returning my body to a state of perfection and healing. Now I would see my entire form radiating out this magnificent healing white light, and I would silently affirm, *"Thank you for my healing, Lord,"* and feel total love and amazing joy for this being true. When I was finished with my "treatment," I would then slowly open my eyes and declare with absolute faith and confidence declare to the universe "I AM

HEALED AND SO IT IS."

Affirm:

"I AM HEALED. LORD, I CANNOT THANK YOU ENOUGH!!!"

LESSON NINE
VisualFestation System Technique:
Scripting

Scripting is another powerful technique which I use frequently during my hour of power. You are essentially writing down what your ideal scene looks like, and what it FEELS like, and giving gratitude for it being true. You always script from the present and NOW, and not from someday in the future (i.e., I AM, not "I will be").

One great way to do this is to imagine you are writing a letter to someone you love, and you are describing all the wonderful things happening in your life. The way I typically do my scripting exercises is to write a thank-you letter to the universe and feel immense gratitude for everything working out perfectly for me.

When scripting, write for as long as the words and the feeling of gratitude flows through you. When you are ready, close the letter and have the feeling that what you have written is DONE and ON ITS WAY TO YOU.

Scripting could also be described as a "written visualization" and should generate the same level of emotion as you do when you have a good day visualizing.

Example:

"Lord, I cannot thank you enough my complete heal-

ing. I cannot tell you enough how great it feels to be enjoying perfect health again. Everyone keeps asking me about miraculous healing. I love being back in my healthy body again and sharing with others how to manifest healing. It is AWESOME beyond words, and I cannot thank you enough for these and all the wonderful blessings which are on their way. THANK YOU SO MUCH!!!"

I have found that scripting works well for me on days which for some reason I cannot get in the "zone" when trying to visualize. Save your journals, as they will be a reminder to you that The **Visual*Festation* System** works, especially when you look back on an earlier page and realize that your healing has HAPPENED and it is now REALITY!!

Affirm:

"I AM HEALED. LORD, I CANNOT THANK YOU ENOUGH!!!"

LESSON TEN
VisualFestation System Technique: Affirmations

Affirmations are written statements which you read aloud to yourself in the present tense. The most powerful statement to begin with and probably the most powerful in the universe is "I AM _____." When you say these powerful words, you are essentially declaring it throughout the universe that it is SO. It is so important to NEVER follow those words with anything NEGATIVE.

What we say to ourselves shapes our beliefs and

our feelings about ourselves. Success is an inside game, we just see the end results showing up on the outside. Often, as adults, we have negative baggage we have carried from childhood which does not support us. If you find your "Self-Talk" sounds like a negative affirmation, put an end to that kind of talk immediately. Remember, whatever you *say* is "Your Truth" shall become "Your Truth."

Example Affirmations:

"I am healed."

"I am a manifester of perfect health in my body and mind."

"I am loved by God and enjoy perfect health."

"I am unstoppable."

"I am living the life of my dreams!"

"I am a co-creator in my experience."

One thing I like to do is write down my affirmations on 3x5 index cards which I carry around with me so I can run through my affirmations during different times of the day. Affirmations are a great thing to read and affirm right before you fall asleep, as they instruct what you want your sub-conscious mind to work on while you rest.

Affirm:

__I AM HEALED. LORD, I CANNOT THANK YOU ENOUGH!!!__"

LESSON ELEVEN
VisualFestation System Technique:
"As If..."

Think, speak, and act "AS IF" is a technique whereby you get into the mindset and feeling of "being," "having," and "doing." You are creating a state of mind in which you feel as if you have achieved your goals, and you create these feelings ahead of the actual event.

One thing you may need to get over is the concept of "make-believe" as something only children play. You live in a world that is "make-believe," and never forget it. Wherever you are in life right now is a result of what you have "believed" and "made."

Example:

Get into the mindset that you are now healed. Start planning that vacation you will reward yourself with as a celebration of your complete healing today. Immerse yourself in the stories of all the other people who have manifested miraculous healing. Knowing that yours is on its way to you, write about your miracle so you can inspire others.

The trick is to get into the mindset of being healed and having perfect health NOW.

Affirm:

"*I AM HEALED. LORD, I CANNOT THANK YOU ENOUGH!!!*"

CONCLUSION

I have provided you with some of the exact techniques my students and I have used to manifest miracles. The physical realm is simply the manifestation of the invisible realm where everything we see is created. The sooner you accept this as fact, the easier it will be for you to manifest whatever you say you want.

Know beyond any shadow of a doubt that the perfect healing is available for you now, and that it is waiting on you to get in to alignment with it. Never allow yourself to buy into any contrary belief.

Remember, there is nothing in this world you

cannot have. It is your birthright. You came here to live the life of your dreams and you have the power inside of you to do just that.

Never forget that you ARE the Genie in the bottle known as your life. You can grant any wish you desire upon yourself, if you are willing to do the necessary work. I wish you Godspeed on your journey, and let us know of your successes so we can inspire others to do the same.

All My Prayers Are With You and I KNOW YOU CAN DO IT!

God Bless,

Pete

To learn more about manifesting miracles, please visit our website at,

http://www.peterdadams.com

where we have a number of resources and products as well as our VisualFestation YouTube Channel where we have our books available as audios which you can listen to for free, and a number of interviews done with Pete.

ABOUT THE AUTHOR

Peter Adams is a philanthropist and both a master and teacher of the Law of Attraction and Manifestation. Pete has studied the greatest teachers of all time, and he has combined their teachings with specific techniques, which he has successfully used to create miracles in his life.

Other books written by the author include *Visu-alFestation: How I Manifested the Life of My Dreams & YOU CAN TOO!* and *The 7 Master Keys for Success with Deliberate Creation: Lessons in Truth for Mani-festing Your Miracles.*

www.ingramcontent.com/pod-product-compliance
Lightning Source LLC
LaVergne TN
LVHW021455080426
835509LV00018B/2288